Food And Disease:

How To Prime Your Body System To Restore Itself

Dr. Vincent McLain

TABLE OF CONTENT

Chapter 1:

Natural Body Restoration system

1. Nerve Recovery

Did you have at least some idea that practical nourishment can assist you with recovering your nerves?

Studies have shown that blueberry, green tea, and carnosine can support immature microorganism recovery in creatures with neurodegenerative illnesses.

Furthermore, spices, for example, ashwagandha, red sage, ginseng, espresso, theanine, lion's mane mushroom, and curcumin, were found to have neurogenic impacts.

2. Liver Recovery

Your liver can likewise recover utilizing a compound known as glycyrrhizin found in licorice. Different substances incorporate oregano, curcumin, Korean ginseng, Vitamin E, and rooibos.

Eating good food varieties, for example, broccoli advances liver capacity and furthermore decreases the aggravation in your blood. Mushrooms are another extraordinary detoxifier for your liver cells.

Moringa separate is another to attempt if your liver requirements security from medications and synthetic compounds.

3. Skin Tissue

The biggest organ of the body is the skin, and it is one tissue that effectively recovers. Ordinary skin recuperating happens at regular intervals, except if the tissue is harmed, then, at that point, it happens all the more rapidly.

We likewise see skin reestablished when we get a cut or scratch, and the body recuperates itself some of the time with scar tissue extra.

Skin answers well to vitamin E, A, B, K, D, selenium, and zinc. It additionally answers well to food sources that contain solid fats.

Food sources that contain good fats incorporate avocados, fish, coconut oil, nuts, and seeds. These can assist your skin with remaining firm, flexible, and saturated.

4. Cardiovascular Cell Recovery

A new examination is at last appearance that the body can recover heart cells. Heart-tissue recovering mixtures are known as neocardiogenic substances.

A portion of these can regrow heart cells, which then, at that point, reestablish sound heart tissue.

Resveratrol, Siberian ginseng, red wine remove, Geum Japonicum, and N-acetyl-cysteine are only a couple of these regenerative heart substances.

Other new examinations show that foundational microorganisms through the placenta can likewise recover heart cells.

You can likewise attempt moringa extra to forestall heart harm and furthermore, increment undeveloped cell creation.

5. Insulin-Creating Beta Cells

Albeit not regularly utilized in the clinical local area, research has shown that a few normal mixtures can recover insulin-creating beta-cells. Solid beta cells are fundamental in switching to diabetes.

Beta-cells get annihilated in insulin-subordinate diabetes. In principle, reestablishing the beta-cells can work on a diabetic's wellbeing to the place where they never again need insulin.

Vitamin D, turmeric, avocado, chard, stevia, goldenseal, unpleasant melon, and arginine are only a couple of the substances that can assist with recovering beta-cells.

6. Chemical Recovery

Chemicals are an indispensable piece of our body's every day work. It is feasible to recover chemicals by expanding the endocrine organs' capacity to emit more chemicals.

L-ascorbic acid, as an enhancement as well as food sources plentiful in L-ascorbic acid, has been shown to help instead of chemical substitution treatment.

7. Ligament Recovery

For those experiencing osteoarthritis, there is trust. Spices and enhancements, for example, Boswellia fish oil, bother, glucosamine, chondroitin, and vitamin E, are only a not many that can work on joint tissue and recovery.

8. Spine Recovery

Like ligament and joint recovery, many enhancements are guaranteed in assisting with the recuperation of a spinal line injury.

They incorporate L-ascorbic acid and vitamin E, as well as marijuana separates and curcumin.

9. Neural Foundational microorganism Recovery

Spirulina is a cyanobacterium that is brimming with supplements. It can assist with immature microorganism creation as well as delay sound cerebrum work.

The coffee berry natural product extricate is another enhancement that can assist with further developing mind action. It might dial back the maturing system that causes pressure.

Like recovery in different regions of your body, curcumin present in turmeric can assist your body with making new synapses. It is additionally notable for decreasing aggravation in your body.

Chapter 2:

Angelic Role Of Gut Tiny Creatures.

How Can It Influence Your Body?

People have developed to live with microorganisms for a long period of time.

During this time, microorganisms have figured out how to assume vital parts in the human body. Indeed, without the stomach microbiome, it would be undeniably challenging to get by.

The stomach microbiome starts to influence your body the second you are conceived.

You are first introduced to microorganisms when you go through your mom's introduction to the world channel.

In any case, new proof recommends that children might interact with certain microorganisms while inside the belly.

As you develop, your stomach microbiome starts to differentiate, meaning it begins to contain a wide range of kinds of microbial species.

Higher microbiome variety is viewed as really great for your wellbeing.

Curiously, the food you eat influences the variety of your stomach microorganisms.

As your microbiome develops, it influences your body in various ways, including:

a) Processing bosom milk:

A portion of the microorganisms that initially start to develop inside infants' digestive organs are called Bifidobacteria.

They digest the solid sugars in bosom milk that are significant for development.

b) Processing fiber:

Certain microscopic organisms digest fiber, delivering short-chain unsaturated fats, which are significant for stomach wellbeing.

Fiber might assist with forestalling weight gain, diabetes, coronary illness and the gamble of malignant growth.

c) Helping control your safe framework:

The stomach microbiome likewise controls how your invulnerable framework functions. By speaking with invulnerable cells, the stomach microbiome can handle how your body answers to disease.

d) Assisting control with brain wellbeing:

New exploration proposes that the stomach microbiome may likewise influence the focal sensory system, which controls mind work.

Along these lines, there are various manners by which the stomach microbiome can influence key physical processes and impact your wellbeing:

1) The Stomach Microbiome Might Influence Your Weight

There are a great many various kinds of microscopic organisms in your digestive tracts, a large portion of which benefit your wellbeing.

Nonetheless, having an excessive number of unfortunate organisms can prompt illness.

An irregularity of solid and undesirable microorganisms is here and there called stomach dysbiosis, and it might add to weight gain.

A few notable examinations have shown that the stomach microbiome contrasted totally between indistinguishable twins, one of whom was corpulent and one of whom was sound. This exhibited that distinctions in the microbiome were not hereditary.

Curiously, in one review, when the microbiome from the hefty twin was moved to mice, they put on more weight those that had gotten the microbiome from the lean twin, in spite of the two gatherings eating a similar eating routine.

These examinations show that microbiome dysbiosis may assume a part in weight gain.

Luckily, probiotics are great for a sound microbiome and can assist with weight reduction. All things considered, studies recommend that the impacts of probiotics on weight reduction are presumably tiny, with individuals losing under 2.2 pounds (1 kg)

2) It Influences Stomach Wellbeing

The microbiome can likewise influence stomach wellbeing and may assume a part in gastrointestinal illnesses like peevish inside condition (IBS) and fiery gut infection (IBD).

The swelling, issues and stomach torment that individuals with IBS experience might be because of stomach dysbiosis.

This is on the grounds that the organisms produce a ton of gas and different synthetics, which add to the manifestations of digestive inconvenience.

Notwithstanding, certain sound microorganisms in the microbiome can likewise further develop stomach wellbeing.

Certain Bifidobacteria and Lactobacilli, which are found in probiotics and yogurt, can assist with fixing holes between gastrointestinal cells and forestall defective stomach conditions.

These species can likewise forestall illness causing microscopic organisms from adhering to the gastrointestinal divider .

Truth be told, taking specific probiotics that contain Bifidobacteria and Lactobacilli can lessen manifestations of IBS .

3) The Stomach Microbiome Might Help Heart Wellbeing

Curiously, the stomach microbiome may even influence heart wellbeing.

A new report in 1,500 individuals found that the stomach microbiome assumed a significant part in advancing "great" HDL cholesterol and fatty oils.

Certain undesirable species in the stomach microbiome may likewise add to coronary illness by delivering trimethylamine N-oxide (TMAO).

TMAO is a substance that adds to obstructed veins, which might prompt respiratory failures or strokes.

Certain microscopic organisms inside the microbiome convert choline and L-carnitine, the two of which are supplements found in red meat and other creature-based food sources, to TMAO, possibly expanding hazard factors for coronary illness .

n any case, different microscopic organisms inside the stomach microbiome, specially Lactobacilli, may assist with diminishing cholesterol when taken as a robiotic.

) It Might Assist with controlling Glucose and Lower the Gamble of Diabetes

The stomach microbiome additionally may assist with controlling glucose, which ould influence the gamble of type 1 and 2 diabetes.

One late review analyzed 33 babies who had a hereditarily high gamble of creating ype 1 diabetes.

t tracked down that the variety of the microbiome dropped out of nowhere before he beginning of type 1 diabetes.

t likewise observed that levels of various undesirable bacterial species expanded ot long before the beginning of type 1 diabetes .

Another investigation discovered that in any event, when individuals were eating recisely the same food sources, their glucose could fluctuate significantly. This night be because of the kinds of microscopic organisms in their guts

5) It Might Influence Cerebrum Wellbeing

The stomach microbiome may even help cerebrum wellbeing in various ways.

In the first place, certain types of microbes can assist with delivering synthetic compounds into the cerebrum called synapses.

For instance, serotonin is an energizer synapse that is generally made in the stomach.

Second, the stomach is genuinely associated with the mind through a great many nerves.

In this way, the stomach microbiome may likewise influence mind wellbeing by aiding control the messages that are shipped off the cerebrum through these nerves .

Various investigations have shown that individuals with different mental problems have various types of microorganisms in their guts, contrasted with sound individuals. This proposes that the stomach microbiome may influence mind wellbeing .

Nonetheless, it's muddled, assuming that this is just because of various dietary and way of life propensities.

Few examinations have likewise shown that specific probiotics can further develop manifestations of gloom and other emotional wellness issues

Chapter 3:

Banish Your Disease, Nourish Your Health

To nourish your health, there are certain meals you ought to take. Taking these meals decreases your chances of coming down with chronic health problems. Examples includes…

1) Eat an assorted scope of food sources:

This can prompt a different microbiome, which is a sign of good stomach wellbeing. Specifically, vegetables, beans and natural products contain heaps of fiber and can advance the development of solid Bifidobacteria.

2) Eat matured food varieties:

Aged food varieties like yogurt, sauerkraut and kefir all contain solid microscopic organisms, primarily Lactobacilli, and can diminish how much illness-causing species are in the stomach .

3) Limit your admission of fake sugars:

Some proof has shown that fake sugars like aspartame increment glucose by animating the development of unfortunate microscopic organisms like Enterobacteriaceae in the stomach microbiome .

4) Eat prebiotic food sources:

Prebiotics are a kind of fiber that stimulates the development of solid microorganisms. Prebiotic-rich food sources incorporate artichokes, bananas, asparagus, oats, and apples.

5) Breastfeed for no less than a half year:

Breastfeeding is vital for the advancement of the stomach microbiome. Kids who are breastfed for something like a half year have more gainful Bifidobacteria than individuals who are bottle-taken care of.

6) Eat entire grains: Entire grains contain bunches of fiber and helpful carbs like beta-glucan, which are processed by stomach microbes to help weight, malignant growth hazards, diabetes and different problems.

7) Attempt a plant-based diet:

Veggie lover diets might assist with diminishing degrees of sickness causing microscopic organisms like E. coli, as well as irritation and cholesterol.

8) Eat food sources rich in polyphenols:

Polyphenols are plant intensifies found in red wine, green tea, dark chocolate, olive oil and entire grains. They are separated by the microbiome to animate sound bacterial development .

9) Take a probiotic supplement:

Probiotics are live microorganisms that can assist with reestablishing the stomach to a solid state after dysbiosis. They do this by "reseeding" it with solid microorganisms.

10) Take anti-infection agents just when essential:

Anti-microbials kill numerous awful and great microorganisms in the stomach microbiome, potentially adding to weight gain and anti-toxin opposition. In this manner, possibly take anti-toxins when medicinally fundamental

Chapter 4:

Ten Remarkable Immune-boosting Meals

1. Citrus natural products

The vast majority go directly to L-ascorbic acid after they've contracted a bug. That is on the grounds that it helps develop your insusceptible framework.

L-ascorbic acid is remembered to expand the development of white platelets, which are critical to battling diseases.

Practically all citrus natural products are high in L-ascorbic acid. With such an assortment to browse, it's not difficult to add a crush of this nutrient to any supper.

Famous citrus organic products include:

1) Grapefruit

2) Oranges

3) Clementines

4) Tangerines

5) Lemons

6) Limes

Since your body doesn't create or store it, you want day by day L-ascorbic acid for continued wellbeing. The suggested every day amountTrusted Hotspot for most grown-ups is:

75 mg for ladies

90 mg for men

Assuming you choose supplements, try not to take in excess of 2,000 milligrams (mg) a day.

Additionally, remember that while L-ascorbic acid could assist you with recuperating from a cold faster, there's no proof yet that it's compelling against the new Covid, SARS-CoV-2.

2. Red ringer peppers

In the event that you think citrus organic products have the most L-ascorbic acid of any organic product or vegetable, reconsider. Ounce for ounce, red ringer peppers contain just about 3 fold the amount of L-ascorbic acid (127 mg) as a Florida orange. They're additionally a rich wellspring of beta-carotene.

Other than supporting your resistant framework, L-ascorbic acid might assist you with keeping up with solid skin. Beta-carotene, which your body converts into vitamin A, helps keep your eyes and skin solid.

3. Broccoli

Broccoli is supercharged with nutrients and minerals. Loaded with nutrients A, C, and E, as well as fiber and numerous different cell reinforcements, broccoli is perhaps the best vegetable you can place on your plate.

The way to safeguard its power is to cook it as little as could be expected - or even better, not in the least. Research from trusted sources has shown that steaming is the most effective way to keep more supplements in the food.

4. Garlic

Garlic is found in pretty much every food on the planet. It adds a little punch to food and it's an unquestionable requirement to have for your wellbeing.

Early civic establishments perceived it's worth battling contamination. Garlic may likewise dial back solidifying of the courses, and there's powerless evidence trusted Source that it assists lower blood pressure.

Garlic's invulnerable supporting properties appear to come from a weighty grouping of sulfur-containing compounds; for example, allicin.

5. Ginger

Ginger is one more fixing many go to in the wake of becoming ill. Ginger might assist with diminishing aggravation, which can assist with lessening a sensitive throat and incendiary sicknesses. Ginger might assist with queasiness also.

While it's utilized in numerous sweet treats, ginger packs some hotness as gingerol a relative of capsaicin.

Ginger may likewise diminish constant pain and could even have cholesterol-lowering properties.

6. Almonds

With regards to forestalling and warding off colds, vitamin E will in general assume a lower priority in relation to L-ascorbic acid.

In any case, this strong cell reinforcement is vital to a solid resistant framework.

It's a fat-dissolvable nutrient, and that implies it requires the presence of fat to be ingested appropriately. Nuts, like almonds, are loaded with nutrient and furthermore have sound fats.

Grown-ups just need around 15 mgTrusted Wellspring vitamin E every day. A half-cup serving of almonds, which is around 46 whole, shelled almonds, gives around 100 percent of the suggested every day sum.

7. Sunflower seeds

Sunflower seeds are loaded with supplements, including phosphorus, magnesium, and the nutrients B-6 and E.

Vitamin E is significant in managing and keeping up with insusceptible framework work. Different food sources with high measures of vitamin E incorporate avocados and dull salad greens.

Sunflower seeds are additionally unimaginably high in selenium. Only 1 ounce contains almost half the selenium that the normal grown-up needs every day.

An assortment of studies, generally performed on creatures, have taken a gander at its capability to battle viral diseases like pig influenza (H1N1).

8. Turmeric

You might know turmeric as a vital fixing in many curries. This dazzling yellow, severe flavor has likewise been utilized for a really long time as a calming in treating both osteoarthritis and rheumatoid joint pain.

Research shows that high groupings of curcumin, which gives turmeric its unmistakable shading, can assist with diminishing activity that instigated muscle harm.

Curcumin has been guaranteed as a safe sponsor (in light of discoveries from creature studies) and an antiviral. More exploration is required.

9. Green tea

Both green and dark teas are loaded with flavonoids, a sort of cell reinforcement. Where green tea truly dominates is in its degrees of epigallocatechin gallate (EGCG), another strong cancer prevention agent.

In investigations, EGCG has been shown to upgrade its safe capacity. The aging system dark tea goes through obliterates a great deal of the EGCG. Green tea, then again, is steamed and not aged, so the EGCG is protected.

Green tea is additionally a decent wellspring of the amino corrosive L-theanine. L-theanine may support the development of microbe battling compounds in your white blood cells.

10. Poultry

At the point when you're wiped out and you go after chicken soup, it's something beyond a self-influenced consequence that helps you to have an improved outlook.

The soup might assist with bringing down aggravation, which could further develop manifestations of a virus.

Poultry, like chicken and turkey, is high in vitamin B-6. Around 3 ounces of light turkey or chicken meat contains almost one-third of your day-by-day suggested measure of B-6.

Vitamin B-6 is a significant player in a considerable lot of the substance responses that occur in the body. It's likewise indispensable to the arrangement of new and sound red platelets.

Stock or stock made by bubbling chicken bones contains gelatin, chondroitin, and different supplements supportive for stomach mending and insusceptibility.

Chapter 5:

Five Mind-blowing Supplements Crucial To Our Being.

1 - L-ascorbic acid

L-ascorbic acid (1,000 mg). Whenever taken in portions of 1,000 mg each day, L-ascorbic acid advances mitochondrial wellbeing essential for cell digestion and other cell capacities.

Likewise, L-ascorbic acid is one of the most well known invulnerable helping supplements accessible, and justifiably it upholds resistant cell creation and multiplication and adds to their usefulness.

At last, L-ascorbic acid is a characteristic cancer prevention agent that decreases your body's development of the responsive oxygen species that cause irritation.

This fundamental reaction can prompt sepsis and untimely cell demise.

2 - Glutathione or N-Acetyl Cysteine

Glutathione or N-Acetyl Cysteine (500-1,000 mg). Known as the most intense cell reinforcement in the body, glutathione offers insurances most others can't coordinate; like L-ascorbic acid, glutathione helps with mitochondria wellbeing for this situation, by keeping harm from free revolutionaries and different poisons.

Likewise, glutathione assists the body with forestalling aggravation. In the mean time, N-Acetyl Cysteine (NAC) has its antioxidative properties and explicitly targets respiratory cells-all while helping your body's glutathione levels.

3 - Vitamin D

Vitamin D (2,000-5,000 mg). When taken routinely, vitamin D forestalls the creation of exorbitant incendiary cytokines and intensifies the microorganism battling capacities of significant white platelets that give your insusceptible reaction.

Research likewise recommends that vitamin D animates peptides that live in your respiratory parcel and assists with safeguarding your lungs against contamination.

Vitamin D is notoriously difficult to get sufficient degrees of, even with a sound eating regimen, so supplementation is critical.

4 - Zinc

Zinc (50 mg). Zinc is probably the best enhancement to support your resistant framework, as it assists your body with directing the creation of incendiary cytokines and has an essential impact in your body's insusceptible reaction to microorganisms.

Likewise, zinc has been shown to explicitly address respiratory lot diseases, shortening their term by a normal of two days. At long last, zinc has various different advantages, including speedier recuperation and worked on mental capacity.

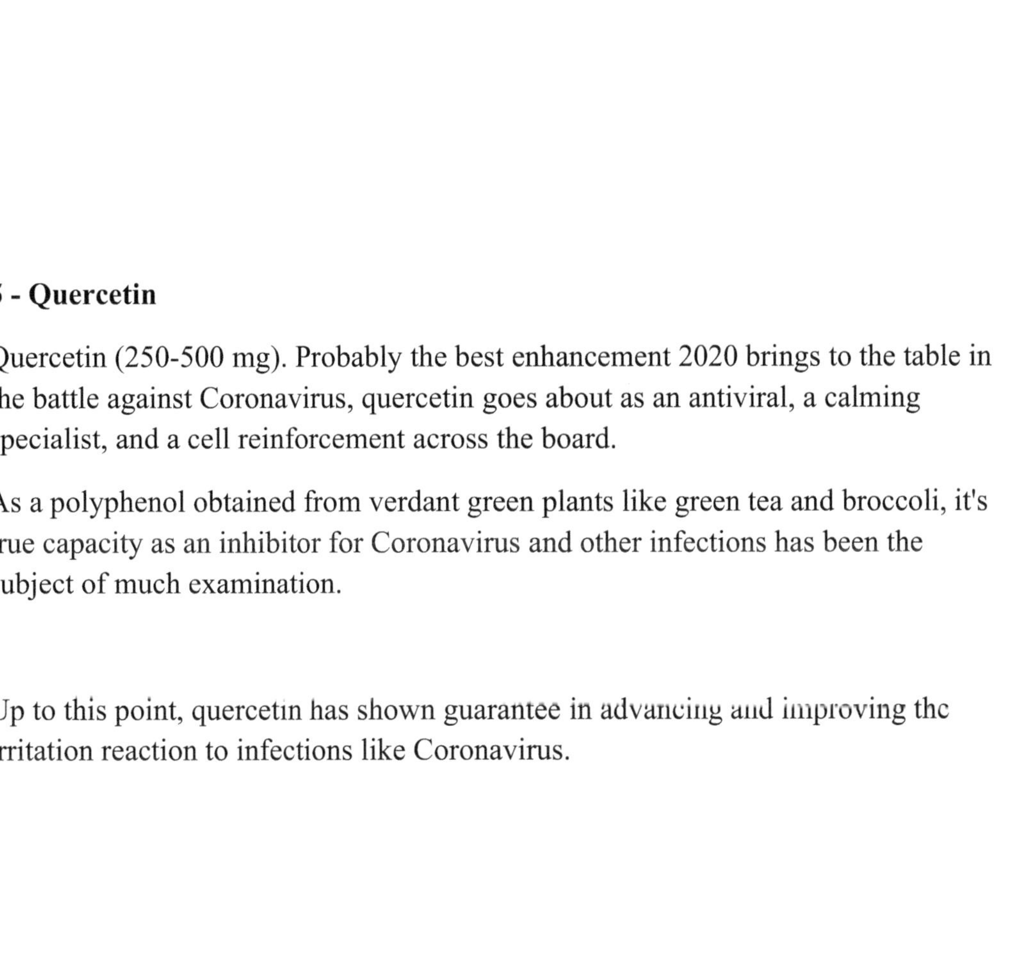

5 - Quercetin

Quercetin (250-500 mg). Probably the best enhancement 2020 brings to the table in the battle against Coronavirus, quercetin goes about as an antiviral, a calming specialist, and a cell reinforcement across the board.

As a polyphenol obtained from verdant green plants like green tea and broccoli, it's true capacity as an inhibitor for Coronavirus and other infections has been the subject of much examination.

Up to this point, quercetin has shown guarantee in advancing and improving the irritation reaction to infections like Coronavirus.

www.ingramcontent.com/pod-product-compliance
Ingram Content Group UK Ltd.
Pitfield, Milton Keynes, MK11 3LW, UK
UKHW022008190726
13853UKWH00004B/1800